AF189699

Gerhard Schumann

Grandma has got Parkinson's

The Parkinson disease made
understandable to children

Gerhard Schumann

Grandma has got Parkinson's

The Parkinson disease made
understandable to children

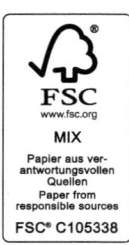

Bibliographic information of the German National Library: The German Library catalogues this publication in the German National Bibliography; detailed bibliographic information can be found on the Internet website: http://dnb.dnb.de.

© 2019 Gerhard Schumann

Co-writer: Moritz Schumann

Manufactured and published by:

BoD – Books on Demand, Norderstedt

ISBN: 978-3-7504-1742-7

Available as e-book

This book belongs to

_____

_____

Content

Introduction

Dear _____!

I'd like to briefly introduce myself.

My name is Gerhard.

I live in Munich, that's a city in Bavaria. Maybe you've already heard about the 'Oktoberfest'. That's the biggest funfair of the world which takes place every year.

And I live nearby.

I live with a woman. Her name is Monika and we are married. I have three children: Sebastian, Florian and Moritz.

When my doctor diagnosed that I had the Parkinson disease, my sons were 4, 13 and 16 years old. Maybe you're aged somewhere in between.

I'm sure you can imagine that Sebastian, Florian and Moritz were quite scared when I told them about my illness.

"I've got the Parkinson disease and there's no cure. I won't become healthy again even if I take pills!"

You probably felt the same when you found out that your Grandma has this disease.

Maybe you've noticed that your Grandma has changed a bit recently and you couldn't figure out why.

With this book, I'd like to explain to you what can happen to someone who has the Parkinson disease. Furthermore, I'd like to show you that you don't have to be afraid of this disease.

Meanwhile I've been living with the Parkinson disease for 10 years and I'm still able to do a lot with my family and friends.

I have to admit though, that in the meantime I started to struggle with some things. However, all in all, we are still leading a normal life, like other families whose Grandma doesn't have Parkinson's.

I hope that with this book I will succeed in answering your questions. I'd like to help you to still spend a lot of nice   moments with your Grandma.

Best wishes from Monika, Sebastian, Florian and Moritz.

Yours

Gerhard

How does the brain work?

First, I'd like to explain to you how the brain works so that you can understand what happens when someone has got Parkinson's.

As you probably know, the brain is in our head. It is a very important and sensitive organ.

Therefore, it's protected by robust bones. The head is also called the skull and the bones are called the skull bones.

In addition to that, there's water between the brain and the skull bones. It works as some sort of shock absorber to soften pushes and shocks.

As the brain is such an important organ, motorcyclists have to wear a helmet.

A lot of people wear helmets while riding a bicycle or skiing to protect their head and brain.

The brain is incredibly complicated and assumes a lot of jobs in our body. Doctors divide the brain in four sections.

These sections are called: the cerebrum, the cerebellum, the brain stem and the interbrain. However, you don't really have to remember this.

Each of these sections has very specific jobs, e. g. speech control, vision control, hearing control and movement control.

There's even a specific place for our feelings in every brain.

Some sections can be trained such as our memory.

Others work all on their own. Our heart is beating without us having to think about it.

Our lungs work automatically too, even when we're asleep.

Furthermore, the brain is divided in two halves: the left and the right brain.

The left brain mostly controls the right side of our body and the right brain controls the left side of our body.

Very smart people took a long time to find this out.

Nonetheless, we don't know exactly how the brain fully works.

Maybe you're going to be the person to research the hidden secrets of the brain one day!

Your muscles need energy to work like a car needs petrol to drive.

Your brain needs energy to fully function. Human beings get this energy by eating food.

Our brain is the switch board or the centre of all vital things happening inside our body.

Here's an example:

Let's say you are not paying attention and you touch a very hot pot with one of your fingers.

What is going to happen?

You will flinch and automatically pull your finger back.

Your brain is taking care of you. It doesn't want you to get hurt and burn your finger.

However, how exactly does your brain protect you?

The skin of your finger, or more precisely the nerve cells receive a certain information:

"Wow, this is very hot!"

They send this information to the brain. Information is constantly exchanged between your brain and your body.

We are not always aware of that.

If there's an information sent to your brain alerting your brain that something dangerous might happen, your brain will ring the alarm bell:

"Attention! Attention! It has just been reported that the finger is moving towards a hot pot. This may cause an injury! The muscles in this section are to move the finger immediately away from this area!"

The muscles react immediately:

"Hello, this is the muscles speaking! We got the finger to safety!"

...that's how it works, approximately.

Neural pathways run through the entire body and exchange information with the brain at great speed.

They exchange information with the muscles in your arms and legs and with your organs such as the heart and liver for example.

However, your eyes and ears are constantly exchanging information.

The neural pathways in our body are comparable to the streets surrounding us.

There are motorways, country roads and 30 zones.

There are buses, lorries, cars and much more on the streets.

Our body doesn't transport goods via these neural pathways, for example like a lorry delivering water to a shop, instead it delivers information.

The doctors call the buses, lorries, cars etc. "messengers".

You can imagine that there's a lot going on in our body, like on the streets surrounding us.

However, a healthy body and brain can handle this without any traffic jams.

If a traffic jam should occur our brain is often able to find a new route and even built new streets.

Sometimes, something goes wrong and then it can happen that we fall ill.

And the doctors' job is to find out what has caused the traffic jam, or why the lorries or cars don't transport the information to the right place anymore.

Furthermore, there are very complicated machines helping the doctors to find the traffic jam.

Very often, the doctors are able to help prevent small or big traffic jams from happening again.

Where does the name 'Parkinson disease' come from?

James Parkinson was a doctor who lived from 1755 to 1824.

He was the first person to do proper research on the disease and wrote down a lot about it.

However, at that time he thought that the disease was some kind of paralysis and therefore called the disease "shaking palsy".

Today we have noticed that the changes have nothing to do with a paralysis.

Although James Parkinson was not entirely right with what he found out, the disease was named after him in his honour.

Maybe you've already heard of the Alzheimer's disease. This disease was also named after its, let's put it that way, discoverer, Alois Alzheimer.

Every year, on the 11th of April, the 'World Parkinson Day' is taking place to remind the people that the Parkinson disease exists.

On this very special day, the researchers explain during numerous events what they have found out recently.

Furthermore, one tries to collect donations, that means money to support the researchers in their work.

What exactly is the Parkinson disease?

Doctor James Parkinson already examined people 180 years ago who were moving peculiarly.

He observed that the patients for example were severely shaking, had difficulties to move or were only able to move slowly.

Researchers have calculated that approximately 500,000 people have the Parkinson disease (alone in Germany!).

Some already know it – they already received their diagnosis – and others don't. Some are still quite young, around 40 years old, and others are already 60 or 70 years old.

Furthermore, researchers think that in the future approximately one out of 180 people will get the Parkinson disease.

In a lot of cases it often takes several years until someone realises that he has the Parkinson disease.

The reason for this lies in the fact that the disease normally progresses very slowly. That means that you don't notice that you're ill and you feel completely healthy.

At some point, the first symptoms appear.

However, it is very difficult for the doctors to diagnose the disease in its early stages. If you have a cold, you've got a runny nose and a cough.

When it comes to the Parkinson disease, there are numerous, very different possible symptoms.

Some think for example, that they have just been working too much and that's why they are often so tired.

Or that they have sat in the office for too long and that's why their shoulders and back are hurting.

Others may think that they've done too much sports.

Or that you are aging and that's why the joints feel a bit "rusty". There are numerous reasons why movements cause pain.

However, people unfortunately get diagnosed with Parkinson's; like unfortunately your Grandma.

Parkinson's is counted amongst the "chronic diseases".

That means that the disease normally can't be cured. However, there is medication for this disease – more on this later.

Until today, no one could find out how the disease occurs and the reason why some people get it and others don't.

One thing is certain: This disease is not contagious. Therefore, it's absolutely not dangerous to give your Grandma your hand or a big cuddle.

Your Grandma can't transmit the disease to you, unlike a cold.

The doctors and researchers assume that it's not a hereditary disease.

You don't need to be scared of getting the Parkinson disease at some point.

The person being diagnosed with Parkinson's has a disease in his or her brain that can't be cured to date.

Of course, that's not great.

However, I'd like to point out again that the Parkinson disease is an illness that progresses slowly.

On the contrary to other diseases you don't have to die from it.

We've already found out that there are many sections in the brain.

One section controls our movements and this section is ill so to speak.

Maybe you already know that the human body consists of many, many, tiny cells.

It's normal that cells die inside the human body, that's true for anybody.

Some cells automatically renew themselves and others don't.

If you've scratched yourself for example and you're bleeding, your body produces cells for the wound so that the wound can heal.

Therefore, the body partially renews itself from time to time over the course of a lifetime.

When you get older, the cell renewal slows down. That's normal as well.

In a specific section of the brain the cells don't renew themselves and die faster than they are supposed to.

Therefore, it's getting increasingly difficult for the brain to control the movements of the body.

And this is what you call the "Parkinson disease".

What might change?

Everyone changes in the course of a lifetime. You grow and get taller; you learn more things and forget others.

You learn how to write at school for example.

In the beginning, that's quite exhausting for you. When you're older and have more practice, it's easy for you and you're able to write quickly without even thinking about it.

When you are writing the brain has to work a lot.

This happens without you noticing it.

Your brain doesn't only have to put the letters in the right order to form the word, but to move a lot of muscles. These little movements necessary for writing are called fine motor skills.

Therefore, it can happen that your Grandma will only be able to write very slowly.

Then, the handwriting is often difficult to read as it's very small and maybe a bit scrawly and illegible.

It's possible that one hand or both hands start to shake at some point.

A lot of people with Parkinson's can't concentrate for a long period of time anymore and get tired more easily.

Maybe you will notice one day that your Grandma's voice has become lower and she's moving more slowly. You can often witness this when somebody is walking.

You might notice as well that your Grandma has a serious look on her face more often and doesn't laugh that much anymore.

That doesn't mean that she doesn't love you anymore!

Everyone has more than 40 muscles in his or her face to laugh. We know by now that the brain won't eventually cope with this that well anymore.

Don't be worried if you notice that. It has nothing to do with you.

There are numerous, different things that gradually become noticeable when the brain cells can't work efficiently anymore.

As there are so many possibilities for the disease to progress and develop, it is called the "disease with 1000 faces".

Parkinson's progresses differently with every patient and the most important is:

Not every Parkinson patient will show all the restrictions.

Furthermore, a lot of research has been done in the meantime and the disease is quite well known.

Therefore, there is a lot of different and good medications to keep the disease well under control for a long time.

You often have to take pills several times a day to provide the brain with the substances it lacks, but your Grandma normally will get used to this quite easily.

A long time later, after years and years, it could be that the pills won't work that well anymore.

If that's the case, there are other possibilities to control the disease. However, this will only be the case much later, maybe in 10 to 20 years' time.

Until then the researchers will probably have had new ideas and found new possibilities to treat that disease even better.

At the end of this chapter, I'd like to tell you that people with Parkinson disease don't automatically become stupid or forgetful.

Although you might have the impression from time to time that your Grandma seems a bit absent-minded or distant, that's down to the facial expression, as you well know now.

I will explain to you later how you can help there.

Do I have to worry about Grandma?

It is a normal, human reaction to worry about someone when you find out that he or she is ill. Especially if you love this person very much and you are very close to him or her like to your Grandma.

Maybe your parents, your grandparents or somebody else that you like very much, have already fallen ill once and had to go to the hospital for a while. Then, you already know how it feels to worry about someone.

However, Parkinson's is not one of those diseases you have to worry about that much.

If someone gets diagnosed with Parkinson's, this news makes them sad at first of course.

Everyone wishes to live long time and be healthy for as long as possible. Most of the people are looking forward to play with their grandchildren and to go on the occasional trip when they have stopped working and are retired.

I've already explained to you that your Grandma probably has to take tablets because of her illness.

She will have to spend some time at the hospital to undertake some "fine-tuning" so that the tablets will work as best as possible.

This "fine-tuning" doesn't hurt. The doctors only try out different sorts of tablets to find the best ones for your Grandma.

Furthermore, these special hospitals offer very good sports and activity programmes so that she will stay strong and mobile for a long time, or so that she will get strong and mobile again. So, if your Grandma has to spend some time in such a hospital, she's well taken care of. They make her feel fit again so that you two can still spend a lot of beautiful moments together.

People with Parkinson's change quicker over the course of time than healthy people.

That means that they will probably get slower, less mobile or just tired a bit more easily. They can grow as old as healthy people though.

Seen from this angle you don't have to be afraid of losing your Grandma quickly.

Can I help Grandma?

Oh yes, you can help your Grandma a great deal and have fun at the same time.

I have already told you that Parkinson's is not contagious, so you don't have to take any precautions when you hug and cuddle your Grandma.

Even a kiss is not dangerous at all.

You can do the same things with your Grandma you've done before she found out that she had Parkinson's.

It is obvious that it's good for everyone to feel loved. I'm sure you feel the same way. However, there are a lot more things you can do with and for your Grandma.

As you already know people with Parkinson's don't feel very bad from one day to the next. It's an "insidious" disease, it's "creeping" slowly.

Therefore, you are able to adjust to the changes and find out which exercises will be good for your Grandma.

I'd like to give you some examples of changes which might occur during the months and years to come and what you can do to slow them down. These are just a few examples.

And you already know: "Parkinson's is the disease with 1000 faces." Not every Parkinson's patient will live through all the changes.

Here we go!

The voice:

The voice can become low and inarticulate.

Exercise:

Make your Grandma read out loud to you as often as possible.

It is especially helpful and funny if she disguises her voice.

For example: As a bear she talks with a really deep voice and slowly, and as a mouse with a high, clear voice and very fast.

Do you have other ideas how to imitate the voices of animals?

The facial expression:

The facial expression only changes slightly or not at all anymore and seems to be somehow frozen.

Exercise:

Make funny faces together until one of you can't help but laugh out loud.

For example: To pull a lemon face, you have to pucker your lips and squint very much as if you have sucked a lemon.

To pull the lion face:

You open your eyes and mouth widely and stick out your tongue as much as you can.

As if you would roar very loudly.

Do you know any other funny faces?

The fingers:

It's getting more difficult to grab things, like to get change out of a wallet.

<u>Exercise:</u>

Try to grab small paper balls with a peg and drop them into a jar, like a digger.

It's fun to compete in this game.

Or you can build a tower out of change.

Don't forget to use different fingers:

Thumb – index

Thumb – middle finger

Thumb – ring finger

Thumb - pinkie

Do you know any other finger games?

Walking:

The steps will become smaller and the sense of balance will decrease.

Exercise:

Try to imitate together the typical way animals walk.

An elephant takes big steps and slumps down his foot.

You can tiptoe like a hunting tiger.

Or you can stand on one foot like a flamingo.

Be careful! Hold on tight to prevent yourselves from falling over.

Which animals have striking and exciting ways of walking?

Big movements:

The movements become smaller and seem stiff.

<u>Exercise:</u>

Use your arms and legs to form the letters of the alphabet and form words that the other one has to guess.

Maybe you can do Yoga or Taiji together.

Throwing a ball is a great exercise as well.

For example: Grab the ball with both hands and throw it like a football player would do from the side line.

Then reverse the process and so on.

Which one of you two is able to throw the ball further and higher?

Training for the brain:

Although the brain is not a muscle you should train it together in order to stay fit for as long as possible.

You are doing that at school, while learning vocabulary for example or learning something by heart.

Exercise:

It's great fun to play the following game: "I packed my bags".

You say the following sentence:

"I packed my bag and in it I put ..." followed by an object, toothbrush for example.

The next player repeats:

"I packed my bag and in it I put the toothbrush..." followed by another object, and so and so on.

It is very helpful to learn phone numbers and addresses by heart.

Maybe you'd like to send someone a postcard and you don't have your address book on you?

"Pairs" is a great game as well.

Do you know it?

My questions and fears!

I left some blank pages for you so that you can write things down.

You've certainly got questions that interest you very much.

Or you are still worrying.

Maybe you don't dare to ask your questions now.

In that case, you can write everything down in this book so that you won't forget them.

Of course, you can write down beautiful and fantastic events.

Anything you like.

Things I'd like to know:

_____

_____

_____

_____

_____

_____

_____

_____

_____

_____

_____

_____

_____

_____

Things that are on my mind at the moment:

_____

_____

_____

_____

_____

_____

_____

_____

_____

_____

_____

_____

_____

_____

Things that I have noticed:

_____

_____

_____

_____

_____

_____

_____

_____

_____

_____

_____

_____

_____

_____

Questions I don't dare to ask at the moment:

_____

_____

_____

_____

_____

_____

_____

_____

_____

_____

_____

_____

_____

Things that have been very funny:

_____

_____

_____

_____

_____

_____

_____

_____

_____

_____

_____

_____

_____

_____

Things I don't want to forget:

_____

_____

_____

_____

_____

_____

_____

_____

_____

_____

_____

_____

_____

Miscellaneous:

_____

_____

_____

_____

_____

_____

_____

_____

_____

_____

_____

_____

_____

_____

The writer

Gerhard Schumann
He was born in 1967 in Munich, is married and has three sons. At the age of 42 he was diagnosed with Parkinson's.
For years, the successful writer has been standing up for the needs and tolerance towards Parkinson's patients.

contact:
buero-schumann@web.de

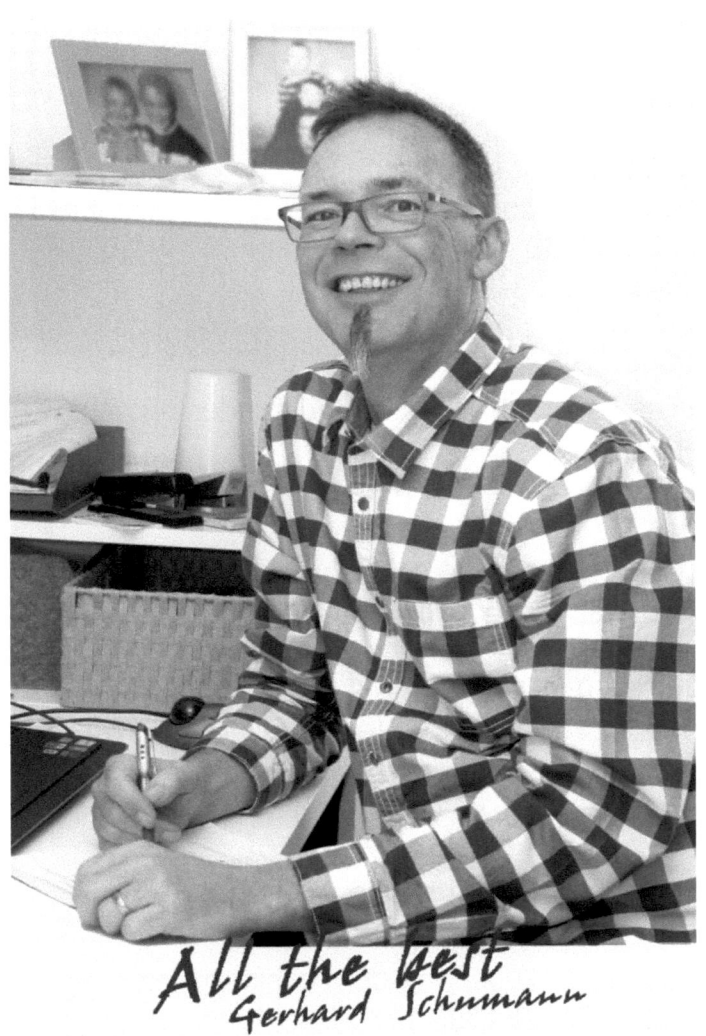

All the best
Gerhard Schumann

Books written by Gerhard Schumann:

<u>Paperbacks:</u>

Dad has got Parkinson´s
The Parkinson disease made understandable
to children
ISBN: 978-3-7504-1010-7

Mum has got Parkinson´s
The Parkinson disease made understandable
to children
ISBN: 978-3-7504-1689-5

Grandpa has got Parkinson´s
The Parkinson disease made understandable
to children
ISBN: 978-3-7504-1743-4

Grandma has got Parkinson´s
The Parkinson disease made understandable
to children
ISBN: 978-3-7504-1742-7

Parkinson Leben mit der Pechkrankheit
ISBN: 978-3-7386-1180-9

Das Parkinson Buch von A - Z
ISBN: 978-3-7412-8423-6

Papa hat Parkinson
Parkinson kinderleicht erklärt
ISBN: 978-3-7322-4717-2

Mama hat Parkinson
Parkinson kinderleicht erklärt
ISBN: 978-3-7481-9295-4

Opa hat Parkinson
Parkinson kinderleicht erklärt
ISBN: 978-3-7481-9275-6

Oma hat Parkinson
Parkinson kinderleicht erklärt
ISBN: 978-3-7481-9393-7

Reich und Berühmt werden
Autorin: Merri Ness / Co-Autor: G. Schumann,
ISBN: 978-3-7431-2771-5

E-Books:

Dad has got Parkinson´s
The Parkinson disease made understandable
to children
ISBN: 978-3-7504-7434-5

Mum has got Parkinson´s
The Parkinson disease made understandable
to children
ISBN: 978-3-7504-7432-1

Grandpa has got Parkinson´s
The Parkinson disease made understandable
to children
ISBN: 978-3-7504-7433-8

Grandma has got Parkinson´s
The Parkinson disease made understandable
to children
ISBN: 978-3-7504-7431-4

Parkinson Leben mit der Pechkrankheit
ISBN: 978-3-7481-2844-1

Das Parkinsonbuch von A - Z
ISBN: 978-3-7481-2846-5

Papa hat Parkinson
Parkinson kinderleicht erklärt
ISBN: 978-3-7494-4439-7

Mama hat Parkinson
Parkinson kinderleicht erklärt
ISBN: 978-3-7494-9326-5

Opa hat Parkinson
Parkinson kinderleicht erklärt
ISBN: 978-3-7494-7646-6

Oma hat Parkinson
Parkinson kinderleicht erklärt
ISBN: 978-3-7494-9329-6

Walddorfer Brudertränen
ISBN: 978-3-7481-2792-5

Herr Hansen
ISBN: 978-3-7392-4539-3

Der Baum von Afrika
ISBN: 978-3-8370-3770-8

Books written by Monika Wimmer-Schumann:

E-Books:

Der kleine Regenwurm Mino traut sich was
ISBN: 978-3-7481-0979-2

Der kleine Regenwurm Mino hilft dem Nikolaus
ISBN: 978-3-7481-1129-0

My special thanks to Karin for the translation!

Contact:

Film 4 Translation
Karin Thorne
karin.thorne@film4translation.tv